Foods You Can Eat If You Have Gout

Home Remedies for Gout That Work to Reduce Pain

By: Doc Goodman

ISBN-978-1493712663

: Foods You can Eat if You Have Gout

TABLE OF CONTENTS

Publishers Notes.. 3

Dedication.. 4

Chapter 1- Foods You Can Eat... 5

Chapter 2- What is Gout?... 6

Chapter 3- Foods Gout Sufferers Can Eat 8

    Complex Carbohydrates.. 9

    Plant Proteins... 10

Chapter 4- Effective Gout Medications 13

Chapter 5- Triggers of Gout Pain 16

Chapter 6- Home Remedies for Gout that Work 17

    Lime... 21

Chapter 7- List of foods to Avoid 24

    Foods to Avoid 26

Chapter 8- Recipes For Gout Sufferers............................... 31

Chapter 9- Final note 37

Doc Goodman

PUBLISHERS NOTES

Disclaimer

This publication is intended to provide helpful and informative material. It is not intended to diagnose, treat, cure, or prevent any health problem or condition, nor is intended to replace the advice of a physician. No action should be taken solely on the contents of this book. Always consult your physician or qualified health-care professional on any matters regarding your health and before adopting any suggestions in this book or drawing inferences from it.

The author and publisher specifically disclaim all responsibility for any liability, loss or risk, personal or otherwise, which is incurred as a consequence, directly or indirectly, from the use or application of any contents of this book.

Any and all product names referenced within this book are the trademarks of their respective owners. None of these owners have sponsored, authorized, endorsed, or approved this book.

Always read all information provided by the manufacturers' product labels before using their products. The author and publisher are not responsible for claims made by manufacturers.

Paperback Edition

Manufactured in the United States of America

DEDICATION

This book is dedicated to All who experience or subjected to this painful disease.

CHAPTER 1 - FOODS YOU CAN EAT

A diet for the individuals with gout isn't necessarily the one which is overly restrictive or unpalatable. Scroll down this Book if you want to know the foods you can eat if you have gout.

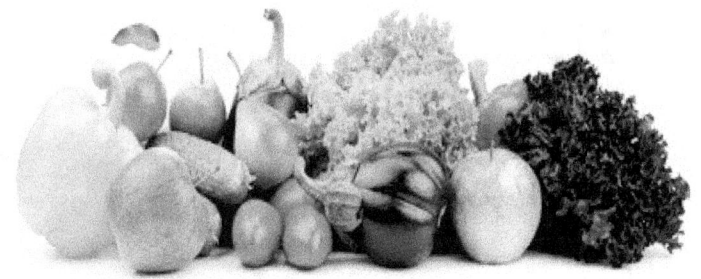

Chapter 2- What is Gout?

Gout refers to a painful form of arthritis causing, stiff, hot and swollen joints. This disorder usually occurs when uric acid builds up in a person's blood. It often effects the feet.
    While the initial gout episodes only may last a few days, the subsequent bouts usually may occur more frequently and end up lasting for longer time periods.

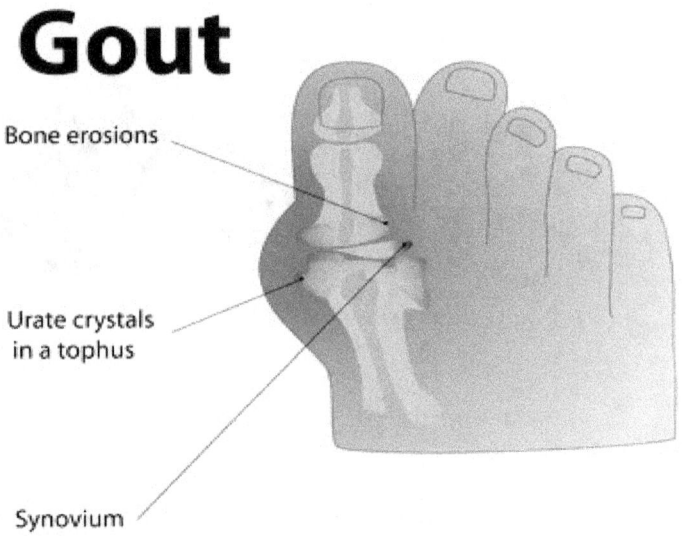

    If gout is left untreated, it can cause permanent joint and liver damage. Fortunately avoiding foods that have high purine levels may alleviate the various gout symptoms in some sufferers. Let us now have a look at the various kinds of food products you should consume if you are suffering from gout.

Doc Goodman

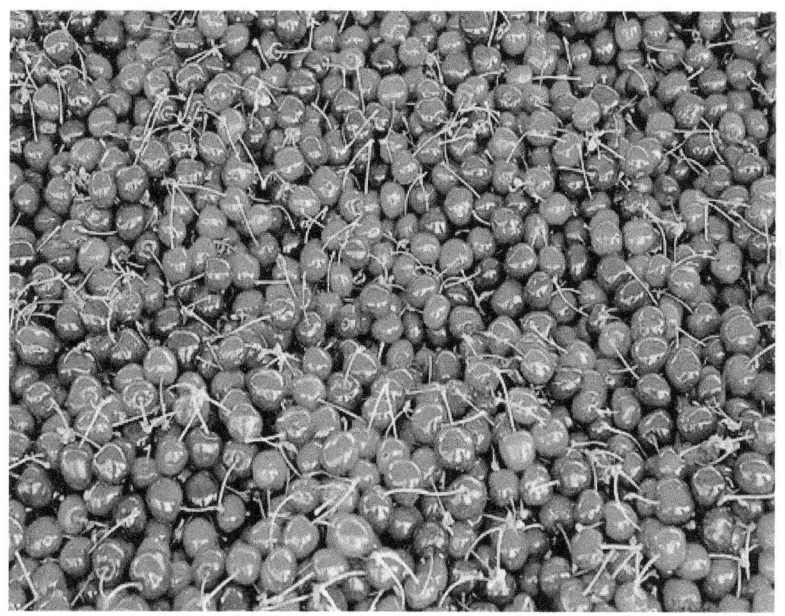

Chapter 3- Foods Gout Sufferers Can Eat

There are certain kinds of foods which can assist an individual suffering from gout. Some of these foods are consumed by gout patients hoping to control the intake of purines. The foods are normally tolerated very well by the body and they do not increase uric acid production to a very great extent.

If you are suffering from gout, here are various **food products that you can eat and** which can greatly contribute to dealing with such a disorder. These food products include:

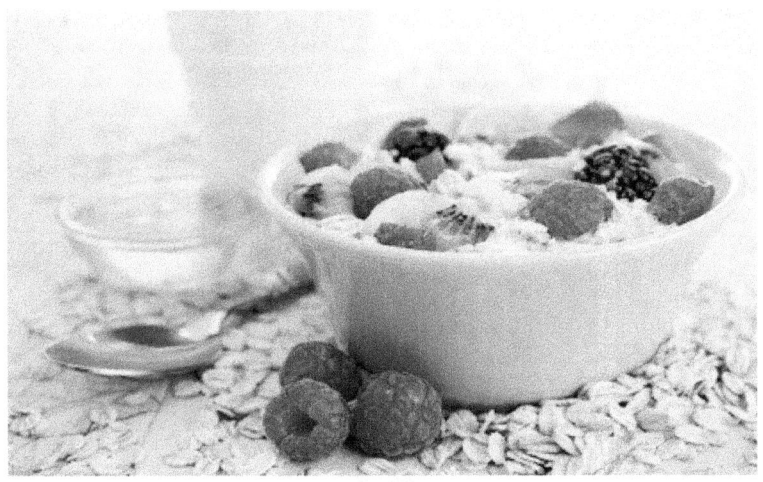

Complex Carbohydrates

Complex carbohydrates can contribute enormously when it comes to assisting gout sufferers. Foods that have high complex carbohydrates levels such as ***potatoes, cereal, cereal products, rice,*** etc. are some of the healthy options which gout patients should add into their diet.

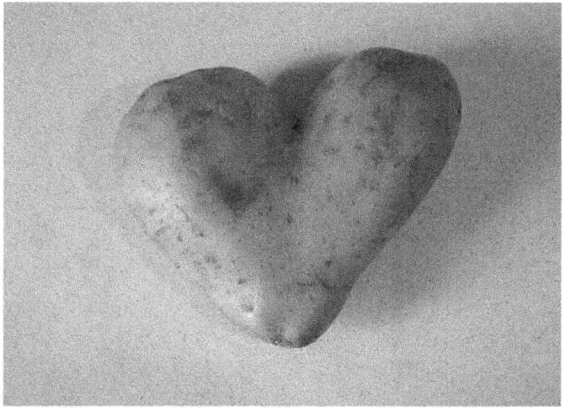

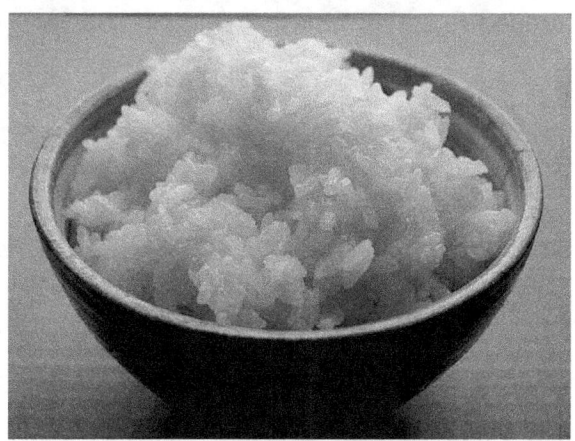

Plant Proteins

Plant proteins can be tolerated very well by the body. Plant proteins are effective when it comes to assisting gout patients since they do not in any way increase uric production.

For an individual suffering from gout, protein intake in the form of plants instead of animal meat is normally advised. Thus, the consumption of peas, beans, mushrooms, legumes, etc. is highly recommended as these food products are very high in protein and thus can assist gout sufferers.

In addition to these kinds of foods, consumption of fresh vegetables and fruits is also a plus point.

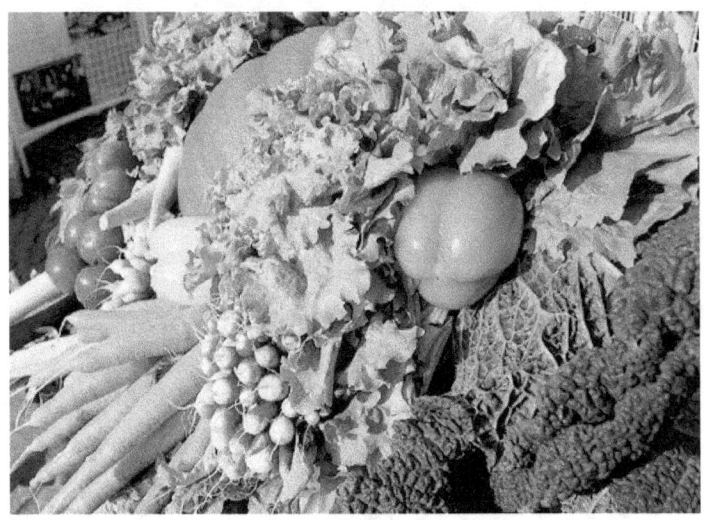

Low Fat Dairy

Foods which have a low amount of fat are also very favorable for the individuals with gout. This is because they assist in reducing the risk of the occurrence of gout. Also, you can drink low fat skim milk or eat low fat dairy products.

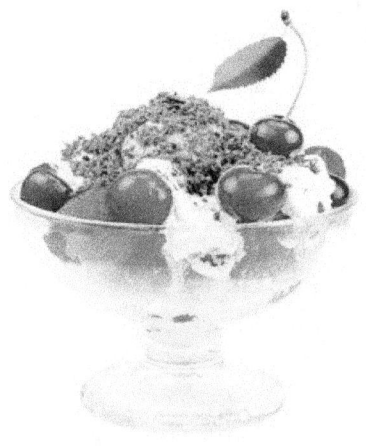

Fluids

If you are a gout sufferer, it is recommended that you always make a point to consume lots of fluids; these fluids should be mostly in the form of juices. Also make a point to drink plenty of water on a daily basis.

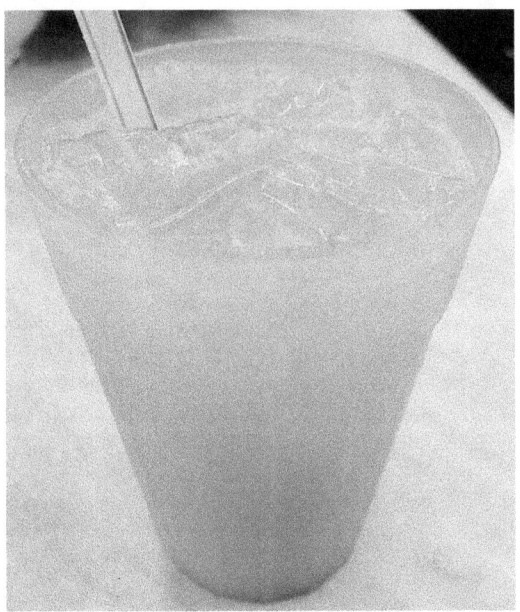

That was a brief overview of the foods which should be included for individuals with gout. Ensure that before you resort to consuming any of the above mentioned kinds of food you consult a physician.

Chapter 4 - Effective Gout Medications

Gout is one of the most challenging ailments. Statistics have revealed that thousands of gout victims suffer silently since they are ignorant about various medications that can be taken in response to gout. Gout can be treated and its treatments involve the use of medicines.

Before opting for any medication, it is advisable that every victim work closely with a doctor or a qualified physician because the choice of medication is dependent on various factors. For instance, before a doctor recommends any particular medication, he/she will have to conduct an analysis of the patient's current health status.

Other factors to consider include the patient's preferences. Which are the most effective gout medications?

Basically, there are several medicines that can be used to treat gout pain. The question is which are the most effective ones? Below find a list of clinically proven medicines that can be used to reverse gout pain.

Non-steroidal

Anti-inflammatory Drugs (NSAIDs)

NSAIDs are some of the most effective gout treatments. They offer help to those who are suffering from various forms of gout including acute gout attack. These forms of drugs have the ability to stop future gout complications in those who use them. The most common varieties that can easily be obtained include; Indocin, Naproxen, Advil and Motrin.

Colchicines

These act as alternatives to NSAIDs and are normally prescribed as a pain reliever. It is the best choice that can be used when symptoms of gout appear. It offers lasting solutions to acute gout attack. Low doses can also be prescribed to prevent attacks in future. It should be given within 48 hours of attacks. These medications should not be used by specific groups of people and therefore it is important to seek a doctor's advice before using them.

Corticosteroids

They control gout pain as well as inflammation. This remedy can be administered in forms of pills or they can be injected into the victim's joints. Ideally, this form of medication is recommended for those who, for any reason, cannot take colchicines or NSAIDs. It should be understood that this medication will subject the user to side effects if not used appropriately and that is why it is advisable to consult a physician before using it.

Xanthine Oxidase Inhibitors

The most essential step in the event of reducing gout pain attacks is to block the production of uric acid. Xanthine Oxidase

Inhibitors like Allopurinol and Febuxostat limits the concentration of uric acid in the body. Lower levels of uric acid will reduce the chances of gout pain.

Probenecid

Probenecid, also called Probalan, enhances the kidneys ability to excrete uric acid that aggravates gout attacks. Once the removal of uric acid is improved, less uric acid will remain in the body and this translates to lower chances of gout attacks.

The bottom line

All the above medications are equally effective However, it is important to use them appropriately to get the best results. Don't forget that there are special guidelines that should be adhered to while using them; never experiment on the medications, always consult a physician.

CHAPTER 5- TRIGGERS OF GOUT PAIN

Aspirin

Diuretics

Dehydration

Extra weight

Fasting

Beer

Menopause

Injury

Uncomfortable shoes

Family history.

To read more on the triggers at the end, in the note page.

Chapter 6- Home Remedies for Gout that Work

Gout is an inflammatory disease which most of the time comes as a form of Arthritis. Actually, around 10% of the people suffering from Arthritis are likely to concede this disease. According to medical researches; gout comes as a result of excess amounts of uric acid in the blood. Kidneys may take too long trying to get the excess amount of uric acid out of the blood.

This will lead to uric acid being deposited in large amounts. Lumpy patches will then start appearing on the skin causing a lot of pain.

The most affected part of the body is the toe and the toe joints. If you are experiencing a lot of pain in your big toe, you may be suffering from gout.

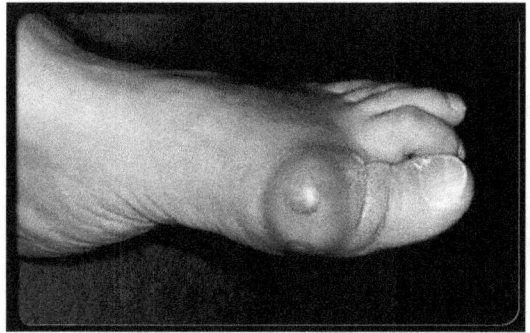

There are many causes for this painful disease that may include consuming a lot of alcohol, eating high purine level foods as I previously mentioned , overeating, and stress among others.

The good news is that it is possible to cure if you take the right remedies. Gout can trouble for years if you do not take necessary measures to cure it.

Some of the drugs that have been introduced only provide relief but they may not cure gout permanently. Some must be taken for a long time before they cure this disease permanently.

The best way to cure gout fast and permanently is the natural way.

Many medical researchers have endorsed the natural remedies as the permanent solution for this disease.

Most of these natural treatment methods are home remedies that almost everyone suffering from gout can start using.

The top home remedies for gout that work include baking soda, mustard powder, lime, apple reserves and cherries

Baking soda

Baking soda is recommended by scientists due its ability to reduce the amount of uric acid in the blood. As discussed above, the main cause for gout is excess uric acid in the blood.

If the amount of this acid can be lowered then the pain caused by gout in the joints will go away. Just mix a spoonful of baking soda in a glass of water and take it.

After about 3 days you should start feeling better. However, make sure you do not take too much of it as it can lead to high blood pressure.

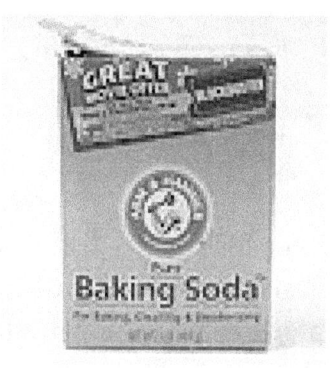

Mustard powder

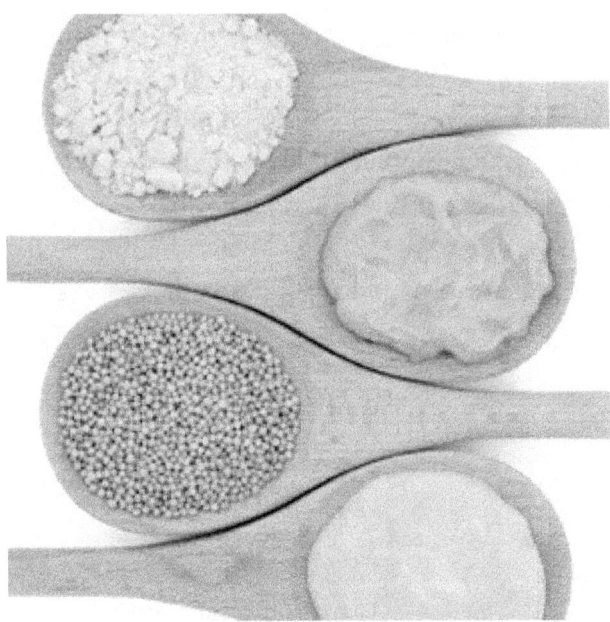

It is usually used as spice for various dishes but it is also a perfect cure for gout. You can start by preparing a plaster of mustard powder. It is simply prepared by mixing mustard powder with a thick paste of wheat flour.

When it comes to applying this paste on the affected area, make sure you start by applying lard or petroleum jelly, followed by the paste using a piece of cloth. The pain will start varnishing within few days.

Lime

Citric acid in lime has the ability to lower the amount of uric acid by neutralizing it, thus reducing the pain caused by gout. Patients suffering from gout are always advised to take lime juice every day in order to reduce the pain

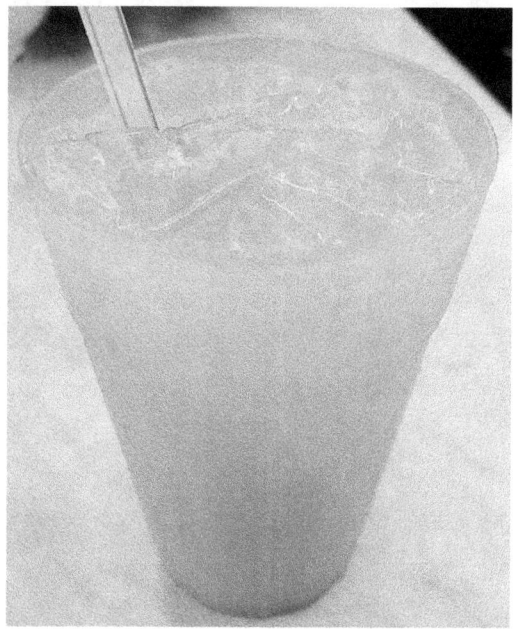

Foods You can Eat if You Have Gout

Apple preserves

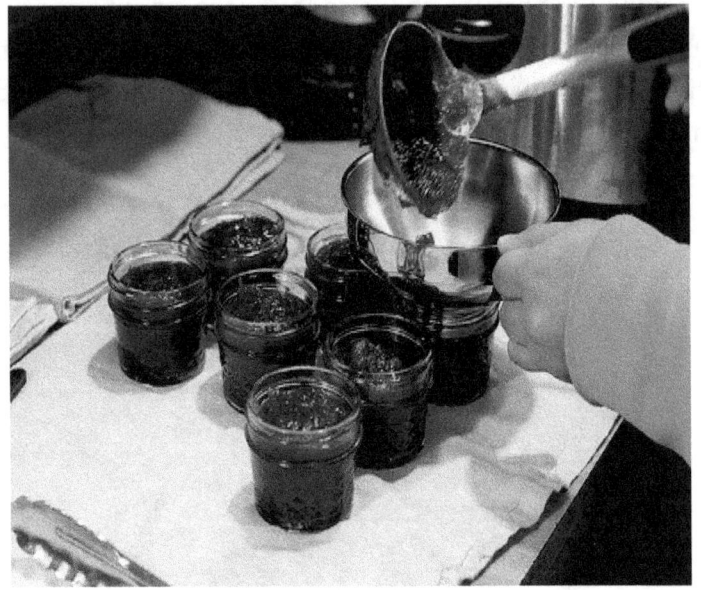

Cherries

Cherries work perfectly in getting rid of toxins from the human body. It can also cleanse the kidneys, giving a complete relief from the pain caused by gout.

This is by far one of the most preferred home remedies for gout that works.

You can have cherry tea, cherry jam or cherry juice. Whichever way you like it, it will definitely provide a cure for gout.

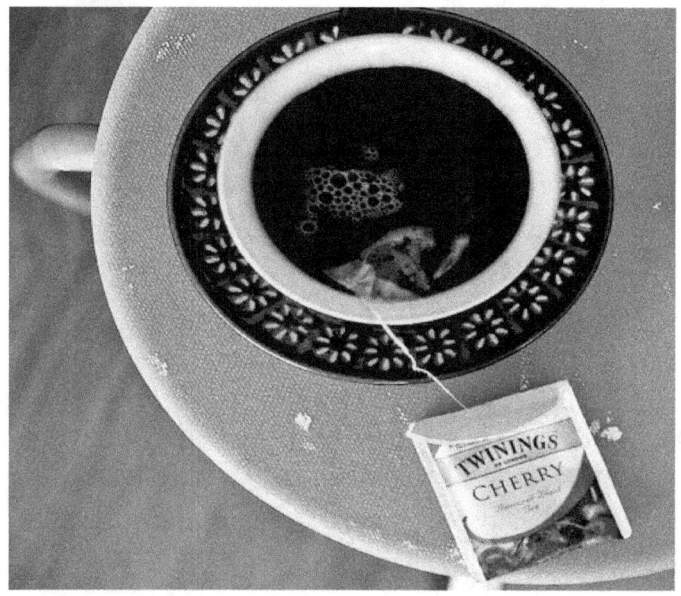

The best thing about these home remedies is that they are readily available and they have no side effects compared to other gout treatment methods.

Chapter 7- List of foods to Avoid

Foods to Avoid with Gout.

Gout is a result of building up of high uric acid levels in the blood. The excess uric acid deposits in the tendons and joints in sharp crystal-like form.

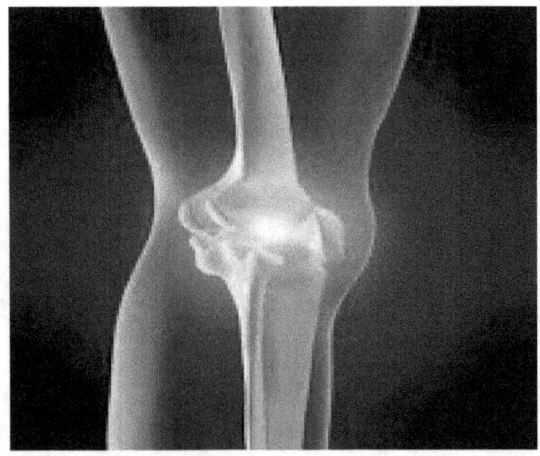

Due to such deposits one suffers from pain and swelling in the affected joints. Excess uric acid can be a result of genetic predisposition, obesity and cancer. It can also result due to improper excretion of uric acid and due to some kind of medications. Certain foods that are rich in purine content also lead to the presence of excess uric acid in the body.

Gout has long been associated with sumptuous meals and is also known as a 'Rich Man's Disease' or ***'Disease of the Kings'***. Purines are the basic link between gout and food. Purines are nitrogenous compounds which are present in the cells of living organisms.

As purines reach the body through dietary resources they are broken down into uric acid, and then through urine are flushed out of the body. Thus, if a person takes in purine rich food in excessive amounts then it can lead to the increase in the amount of uric acid present in the blood and thus trigger gout. So to deal with gout you need to limit your intake of food rich in purines and if you are already suffering from gout, then you should avoid such food items as much as possible. Below is given a list of foods you need to avoid with gout.

FOODS TO AVOID

There are certain vegetables that you need to avoid if you are suffering from gout. You need to remember that the exact food item that causes gout differs in different people, so you will need to do some experiment to find out which of these vegetables affects your condition. Legumes, peas, mushrooms, lentils, asparagus, cauliflower and spinach are amongst vegetables that you need to avoid since they are quite rich in purines. You can however have them in very limited quantities.

Most meats, including fish and poultry are rich in purines, so you need to avoid them if you suffer from gout. If you like having meat then have it in very limited quantity, particularly the meats that have high levels of purines like mackerel, organ meat (liver, heart), anchovies and herring.

Red meats and certain fish like salmon, tuna, lobster, cod, shrimp and scallops have moderate to high purine content. Poultry, like turkey, chicken and pheasant can also cause gout attack. You should not consume more than six ounces of these purine rich foods on a daily basis.

Though not a food, alcohol is still worth a mention in the list of foods to avoid, since it greatly reduces the uric acid elimination. Beer needs to be avoided completely as it can easily trigger gout attacks.

Dairy products rich in fat content also needs to avoided if you are suffering from gout. It will be best if you opt for low-fat or better still fat-free dairy products. According to some research, certain dairy products like skim or low-fat milk and yogurt actually help minimize the chance of a gout attack.

Many foods that you need to avoid with gout are protein rich food and your body needs protein to remain healthy. So, if you are following a gout diet, do keep a check on your protein intake, and if required, eat some low purine protein rich food or include some other sources of protein in your diet like protein powders or protein bars.

Foods You can Eat if You Have Gout

As a form of arthritis, gout is usually controlled with a proper diet. If you indulge in alcohol, red meats and some seafood, uric acid develops in your body, causing joint inflammation.

Crystals actually pack around your joint to cause mobility problems and pain. Several food and recipe choices reduce your joint pain without using daily painkillers.

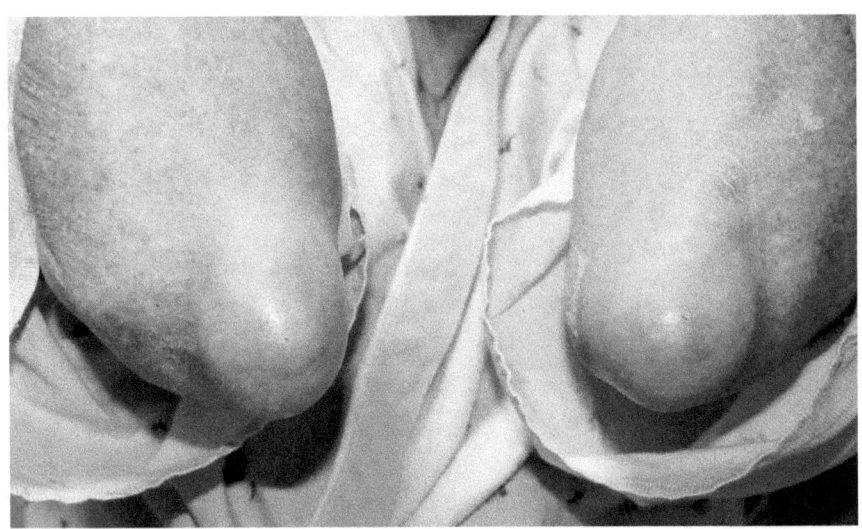

Foods To Avoid as I mention above

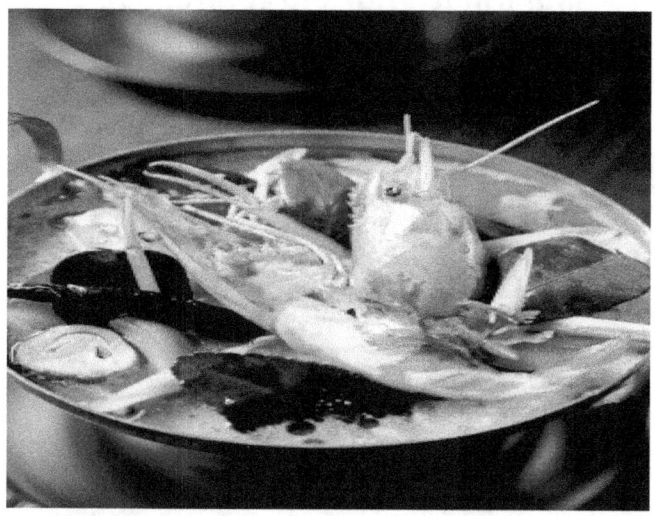

Organ meats, anchovies and some shellfish should be avoided, along with meat portions larger than 6 ounces each day. Purines in the meat must be broken down, causing uric acid to fill your joints and inflaming gout. Alcohol, especially beer, needs to be moderated or eliminated altogether.

Concentrate on natural fruits vegetables and whole grains to control gout.

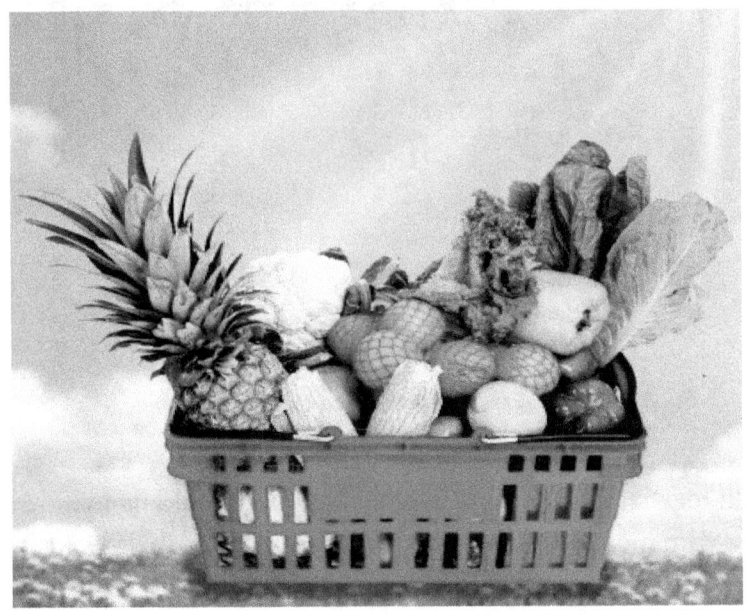

CHAPTER 8- RECIPES FOR GOUT SUFFERERS

Vegetable Soup Recipe

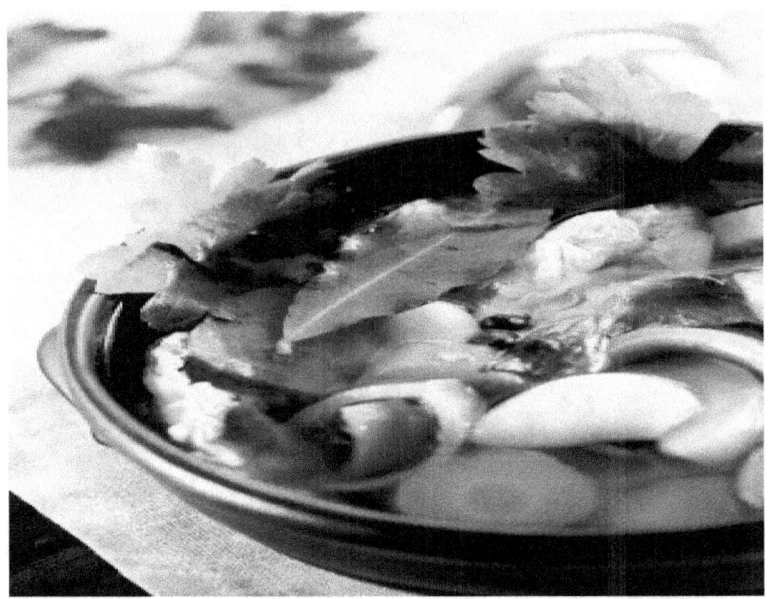

Combine diced potatoes, tomatoes, garlic, onion, carrots and ginger in a slow-cooker pot. Season the vegetables with cilantro, cayenne pepper, black pepper, cumin and a pinch of salt.
You want to use as little salt as possible and increase flavor with spices to reduce gout pain.

Cover all the vegetables and spices with water. Cook on low for 4 to 6 hours. You should have a rich vegetable soup that satisfies your appetite.

Taco Salad

Boil chicken breasts and saute them with onion, tomato, cumin and chili powder. Using pre-made taco salad shells, line the interior with shredded lettuce. Spoon the sauteed chicken mixture into the shell. Add avocado, sour cream, cheese, olives and salsa on top. Along with gout-friendly ingredients, you also have a complete meal with protein, grains, fruits and vegetables.

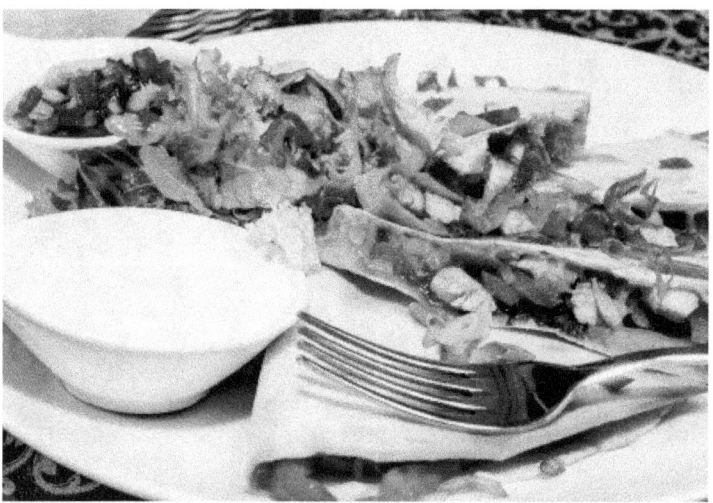

Chicken With Noodles

Boil fettuccine noodles until al dente. Combine the noodles with Parmesan cheese, pepper, garlic, coriander and olive oil. Boil chicken breasts until cooked thoroughly. Shred the chicken and mix it into the noodles. You have a comforting meal for a cold day.

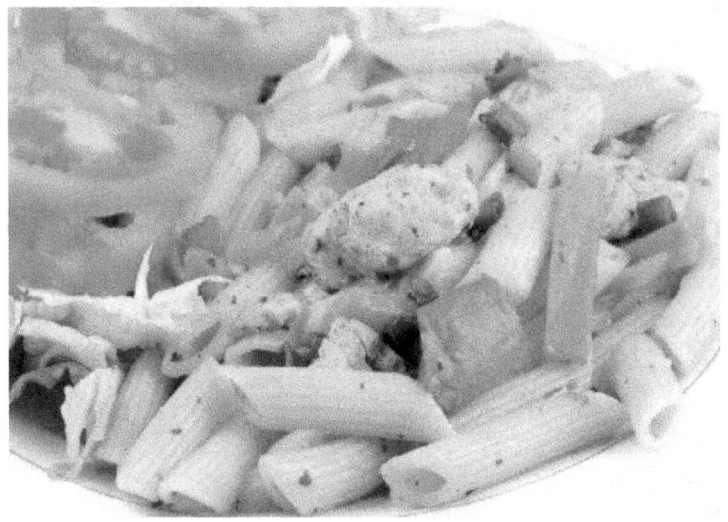

Yogurt Dessert Treat

Blend your favorite flavor of yogurt with water using a 5:2 ratio. Pour the mixture into cups and add crushed ice. This smoothie alternative provides critical dairy nutrition along with beneficial bacteria found naturally in the yogurt.

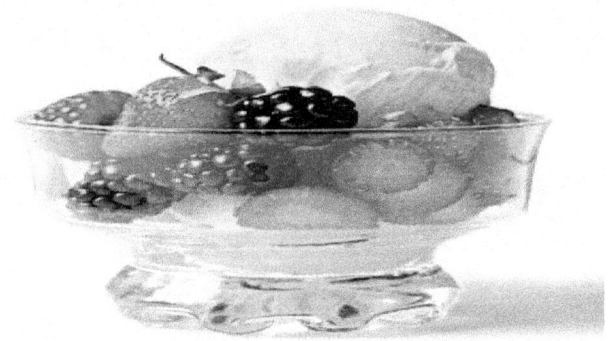

Gout does not have to be a debilitating joint disease. Analyze your eating habits and create recipes with some of your favorite foods. Some of the most common foods, such as beef hamburgers, can be substituted with different ingredients, including ground chicken or turkey.

Keep an open mind and you may find that alternative foods are more satisfying than high-purine meats, seafood and alcohol.

CHAPTER 9- FINAL NOTE

As you can tell this book is a guide on what to do when suffering from gout.

You can be your own physician, but it is always a great idea to consult with your health care provider.

To read more on the triggers of gout pain

health.com

All the best, stay healthy!
Doc Goodman

www.ingramcontent.com/pod-product-compliance
Lightning Source LLC
Chambersburg PA
CBHW070725180526
45167CB00004B/1615